Hyperventilation Syndrome

A HANDBOOK FOR BAD BREATHERS

Dinah Bradley

Illustrations by Sally Hollis-McLeod

KYLE CATHIE LIMITED

Dinah Bradley is a New Zealand trained and qualified physiotherapist who during twenty years of practice has worked in Britain, Australia and New Zealand. She has been involved in many areas of health care including childbirth education, geriatrics, neurology and respiratory medicine and has also worked as a freelance writer, photographer, TV researcher and women's health activist.

Her published works include *Grandma's Teeth*, a picture book for children, *Becoming Single,* which she co-wrote with Hamish Keith, as well as editing the New Zealand edition of *Women's Health* by Sandra Cabot.

Dinah Bradley lives in Auckland with her husband and two teenage sons.

First published by Tandem Press, New Zealand in 1991

First published in Great Britain in 1994 by
Kyle Cathie Limited
7/8 Hatherley Street, London SW1P 2QT

ISBN 1 85626 166 2

A Cataloguing in Publication record for this title is available from the British Library.

Illustration by Sally Hollis-McLeod
Typeset by Books Unlimited (Nottm), Rainworth, NG21 0JE
Printed in England by Cox & Wyman, Reading

Contents

Acknowledgements

Grateful thanks to Helen Benton and Bob Ross for their enthusiasm and decision to publish this book.

Heartfelt thanks, too, to John Henley for his help and encouragement, and to my physiotherapy colleagues.

I would like to acknowledge research material by British physiotherapists A. Pilgrim and Diana Innocenti, and the brilliant literature by chest physician L. C. Lum, MA, MB, FRCR, FRACP, and P. G. F. Nixon, FRCP, whose clear and in-depth views were so valuable and inspiring.

Special thanks to Sally Hollis-McLeod for her superb cartoons.

Finally, I must mention the many patients who helped me experiment, formulate and shape the BETTER breathing programme, especially Rosa, who goaded me into producing this book.

Dinah Bradley

Foreword to the British Edition

The newly graduated doctor, bursting with the latest medical science, soon finds that this science has not equipped him to cope with the illnesses of a third of patients seeking his help. He resorts to a flurry of expensive but fruitless investigations, ends up confused, angry at his own impotence and often dismisses the patient as neurotic.

For most of this century English medicine, with few exceptions, has turned its back on this problem. The notable exception was the great English physician, Sir Thomas Lewis, who in 1921 showed that these varied illnesses shared a common factor which we now know as a hallmark of hyper-ventilation.

By 1940 he declared it to be the commonest disease afflicting civilised society. At about the same time an eminent American research team were writing, 'Patients presenting the well-known pattern of symptoms haunt the offices of physicians and specialists in every field of medical practice. They are often shunted from one physician to another, and the sins of commission inflicted upon them fill many black pages in our book of achievement.'

It is only now, half a century later, that the situation is beginning to change. Coincident with the launch of this book, the newly formed International Society for the Advancement of Respiratory Psychophysiology (ISARP) will be having its inaugural meeting in Saint-Flour, France.

Delegates and members will be the many doctors, therapists and researchers from America, Canada, Europe and Great Britain who over the last fifteen years have shared a common interest in hyperventilation and its effects on human behaviour and well-being.

Thirty years' work within this field has convinced me of the truth of Sir Thomas Lewis' observations. Hyperventilation is a major factor in the 'stress' illness afflicting the modern world.

Dinah Bradley's timely book will bring relief and hope to the many sick people who find their illness baffles, and often irritates, their physicians. These are the patients at whom this book is aimed. Its admirable blend of knowledge, clinical experience and readability not only tells patients what is wrong with them, but also shows that something can be done about it. The book rapidly became a bestseller in New Zealand and Australia. I wish it similar success here.

Dr. L. C. Lum MA, MB, FRCP, FRACP
Emeritus Consultant in Chest Medicine and Respiratory Physiology, Papworth and Addenbrookes Hospital, Cambridge, and ex-Vice President of the Royal Society of Medicine

Foreword to the New Zealand Edition

In the Western world we are suffering from
what has been called the paradox of health.
Despite the fact that collective health has
improved dramatically, perhaps because of
technological advances and concentration upon
preventative measures, there is a declining
satisfaction with personal health. Many people
report disturbing somatic symptoms and feelings of
general illness.

One of the major reasons is the widespread
commercialisation of health and the media's
increasing focus on health issues, creating
apprehension, insecurity and alarm about disease,
real or imagined.

A major result of such tension is the condition of
chronic hyperventilation, or Hyperventilation
Syndrome. Although known about for many years,
it has been largely ignored as a diagnostic
alternative, resulting in extensive investigations that
heighten the patient's anxiety. A bewildering
collection of seemingly unrelated symptoms can be
provoked by this condition, and recognition of its
presence by health professionals is important, not
only because reassurance can be given, but
treatment is simple and usually very effective.

Dinah Bradley in this monograph has beautifully
presented the symptoms of Hyperventilation
Syndrome and the therapy options available.
Her book is very timely, as it seems more
important now than ever to prevent extensive

and expensive medical investigations and to get patients back to feelings of good health. Above all, it highlights the need for health professionals to have better communications with patients, to understand their fears and anxieties, and to help them conquer these.

This book will not only be appreciated by thousands of patients who will recognise themselves in its pages, it will also be very helpful to all those looking after the chronically ill. I wish it the success it deserves.

John Henley, MB, ChB, FRACP

Introduction

'It's as easy as breathing' is a common enough expression.

But for a great number of normal people, breathing is not easy.

They experience an increased drive to breathe, sometimes quite unconsciously, which leads to a chronic health disorder that can be both frightening and mystifying. Called Hyperventilation Syndrome (HVS) it's a widespread cause of ill-health today which remains largely unrecognised.

Short-term over-breathing is a normal reaction to sudden stressful events. Human beings are designed to cope well with these. Normal breathing returns when the fear or danger is over. But many of our present-day stresses are far from short-term.

Worries over jobs, health, security, isolation or violence — the essence of life in the 1990s — seldom go away after a good night's sleep. In fact these prolonged anxieties lead to broken sleep — and exhaustion. If this goes on for too long, it's likely to become habitual. The very unpleasant, baffling, sometimes devastating symptoms which result can fool you and your doctor into thinking you have a serious disease.

'If there's nothing wrong with me why do I feel so wretched?' is another common cry many doctors hear as yet another patient receives the good news that their tests are all normal.

Desperate sufferers may then seek alternative health care with more bank-breaking bills and bizarre diagnoses, further cranking up anxiety levels. But the basic problem — breathing dysfunction — is not being diagnosed or treated.

And then there are those who already have chronic disorders, such as asthma, arthritis or heart disease. Natural anxieties are often made worse if disordered breathing (and resulting upset body chemistry) adds to the problem.

After reading through this book — it's designed to be read at a sitting — draw up a plan for yourself. Place in order the things that need attention, and discuss the plan with family and friends. Remember, there is no 'quick cure'. Don't be discouraged. Allow time and patience to recover, regain equilibrium and confidence, while you practise BETTER breathing.

One

What is hyperventilation?

Hyper=too much, excessive, over the top.
Ventilation=the flow and movement of fresh air.

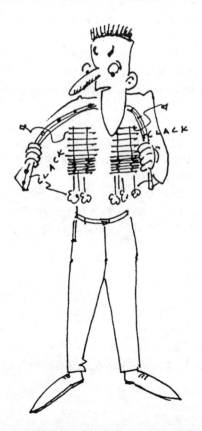

Hyperventilation Syndrome

Hyperventilation means using the lungs to move more air in and out of the chest than the body can deal with.

Most people have experienced this in the short term. It's a normal reaction to a wide variety of events that stress or frighten people. It may be triggered by sudden exertion, such as jumping out of the way of a speeding car, or fear (sitting exams or going to job interviews) or intense emotions, such as love, rage, pain or tears.

The body becomes primed for action.

- Adrenalin pours into the bloodstream.
- Heart and breathing rates speed up.
- Muscles become tense.
- Eyesight and hearing sharpen.
- Pain thresholds drop and pain is less intense.

Usually, when the danger or stress is over, the body returns to a relaxed state with normal heart and breathing rates.

But for some, over-breathing becomes a habit. When this happens frightening and widespread symptoms are commonly experienced.

- Erratic heart-beats and/or chest pain.
- Breathless 'attacks' at rest, for no apparent reason.
- Frequent sighing and/or yawning.
- Irritable coughing and chest tightness.
- Dizziness and 'spaced out' feelings.
- 'Pins and needles' or numbness in lips, fingertips and toes.

• Gut disturbances — indigestion, nausea, wind or
'irritable bowel'.
• Muscle aches, pains or tremors.
• Tiredness, weakness, disturbed sleep and
nightmares.
• Phobias.
• Clammy hands, and feelings of high anxiety.
• Sexual problems.

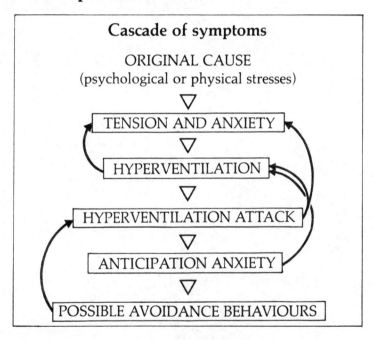

Cascade of symptoms

ORIGINAL CAUSE
(psychological or physical stresses)
▽
TENSION AND ANXIETY
▽
HYPERVENTILATION
▽
HYPERVENTILATION ATTACK
▽
ANTICIPATION ANXIETY
▽
POSSIBLE AVOIDANCE BEHAVIOURS

Many cultures exploit controlled hyperventilation
— before battle or competition or during religious
festivals to induce trance. New Age psycho-
therapy techniques such as rebirthing — where
people are asked to overbreathe for long periods —
use it as a therapy. A study using two groups of
students explains why, with a positive

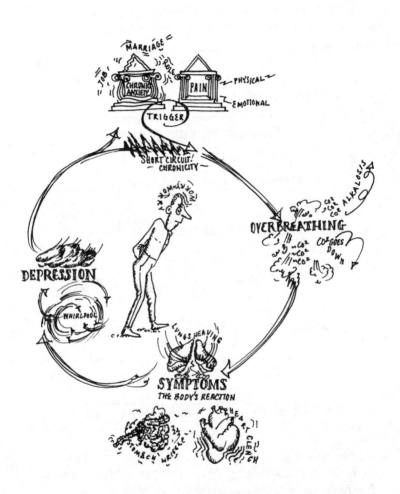

outlook, hyperventilation might be felt as beneficial. Members of the first group were told they would experience faintness and tingling, when they hyper-ventilated, indicating 'heightened consciousness'. They found the experience pleasurable. The second group was told that their over-breathing may lead to collapse. This group understandably became anxious.

Prolonged, habitual or chronic hyperventilation, however, is a thoroughly unpleasant disorder and can become disabling.

How does this happen?

The exchange of air we breathe in (oxygen) and air we breathe out (carbon dioxide) is balanced by the lungs.

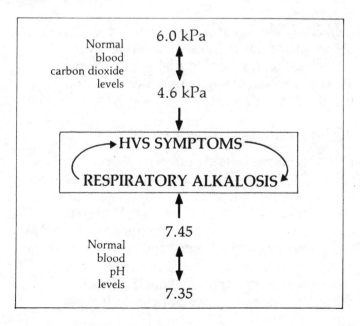

Hyperventilation upsets this vital balance because more carbon dioxide is breathed out than normal, and carbon dioxide levels in the blood start to drop. This upsets the normal acid/alkaline balance (pH) of the blood, and as a result the body becomes more alkaline than normal. Nerve cells are the first to respond to this state of respiratory alkalosis. Dizziness, 'pins and needles' or numbness are usual first signs.

If carbon dioxide levels in the blood fall further with continued overbreathing, body cells begin to produce lactic acid in an effort to balance the body's pH and reduce the alkalosis. Metabolism is less efficient. Exhaustion and chronic tiredness soon follow, with feelings of physical and mental depression — all typical signs of Hyperventilation Syndrome.

In a terrible Catch 22 cycle, natural anxiety about symptoms increases the tendency to over-breathe, further increasing respiratory alkalosis, which leads to more unpleasant or frightening symptoms.

All systems are affected

Not only nerve cells are affected. Smooth muscle cells are galvanised into action by lowered carbon dioxide levels, which leads to tightening or constriction of the blood vessels. The heart and pulses start pounding, and the hyperventilator may feel panic-stricken with palpitations and chest pain. The brain may have its oxygen supply cut by as much as 50 per cent, making it difficult to think, or concentrate, let alone even feel part of this planet. Ultimately, all systems in the body are affected, leading to a puzzling constellation of symptoms.

Carbon dioxide, far from being just a 'waste gas' at the end of the respiratory cycle, is actually a powerful governor of many of the body's functions. It is also the chief controller of the diameter of the blood vessels supplying the brain.

Why does this happen?

Everybody reacts in different ways to daily stresses and strains. For many people, life in the 1990s has been full of change and uncertainty. Adapting to change often brings with it anxiety, especially if the changes are unwanted as happens in marriage break-down, money worries, failure at school or redundancy. Feelings of helplessness and loss of personal control over events, even relatively small things, can corrode self-esteem and confidence. Anxiety levels soar higher, and with them adrenalin levels, heart rate and nervous tension — all fuelled by overactive lungs.

Is hyperventilation a new syndrome?

Over the centuries many observations have been made about 'the breath of life'. Hippocrates, the 'father of Western medicine', in the fifth century BC noted: 'The brain exercises the greatest power in mankind . . . but the air supplies sense to it.'

Buddhism, which originated in the fifth century BC

in India, had detailed accounts of breathing techniques to sustain health. These methods spread throughout Asia, and are best known in the twentieth century as yoga.

In ancient China Taoism also had respiratory physio-therapy methods that combined breathing with relaxation and exercise to harmonise the various body systems, such as heart rate, circulation, digestion and breathing. Movement and rest were evenly balanced. (The Chinese word for the interaction of exercise and rest literally translates as 'feeding'.)

Apart from well-observed accounts of swooning heroines and thunderstruck heroes in seventeenth- and eighteenth-century literature, little was understood about the link between over-breathing and ill-health in the West. Florence Nightingale, the 'mother of nursing', was told she had heart disease when she suffered chest tightness, pain and anxiety, and lived the latter half of her life as a semi-invalid. That she lived until she was 90 years old makes it unlikely that heart disease was her major problem.

Scientific medical history

The first detailed medical account of this syndrome was published in 1871.

Known as Da Costa's syndrome, it was named after the doctor who had recorded his studies of 300 soldiers during the American Civil War. He pinpointed their 'disabling shortness of breath and irritable heart' and the 'oppression' of breathing, and thought that the source of the problem lay in the heart.

By the First World War the condition was commonly known as 'soldier's heart'. American doctors working with the British Medical Corps rejected this name, partly for psychological reasons but mainly because signs of true heart disease were rarely found.

Some soldiers discovered a method of mimicking the syndrome's symptoms (not realising that a few minutes' heavy breathing would have done the trick) by ingesting gunpowder, or 'biting the bullet', in an attempt to escape from the horrors of war. This risky method was soon replaced by a much more permanent escape — death by firing squad — if soldiers were caught with gunpowder on their breaths.

Sir Thomas Lewis, a physician who coined the terms 'soldier's heart' and 'effort syndrome' in the 1920s, described the syndrome as 'one of the commonest chronic afflictions of sedentary town-dwellers'.

Further research in the 1930s and 1940s increased knowledge about the physiology behind Hyper-ventilation Syndrome, but emphasis was still on it being secondary to primary neurotic or anxiety disorders ('the vapours'). Breathing into a paper bag (rebreathing exhaled carbon-dioxide-rich air) became a popular treatment for acute attacks of hyperventilation. No theatre would be without a paper bag in the wings for stage-fright victims, frozen in respiratory alkalosis (terror) before making their entrance.

While still widely used in the treatment of acute 'panic attacks', the paper bag technique is, however, of no use to habitual hyperventilators because it fails to correct the basic cause — disordered breathing. It also makes chronic hyperventilators dependent on something outside themselves — a crutch they might panic over being without.

Note: It can be extremely dangerous if those with acute asthma panic and try to control their rapid wheezy breathing in this way. An increased respiratory drive is normal during an attack. At least one person during a severe asthma attack is on record as breathing their last breath into a brown paper bag.

Opinion is still divided today as to the true origins and definitions of Hyperventilation Syndrome. One camp treats the psyche first and lets the breathing take care of itself; the other emphasises retraining of breathing rate and pattern (and rebalancing blood gases) and letting the psyche take care of itself.

This book attempts a combination of both approaches.

Further reading

The Chinese Art of Healing, Stephen Palos (Bantam Books, New York, 1972).

From Medicine Man to Freud, Jan Ehrenwald (Dell Publishing, New York, 1956).

'Hyperventilation Syndrome: Infrequently Recognised Common Expressions of Anxiety and Stress', Gregory Margarian, *Medicine*, vol. 64, no. 4, 1982.

'Hyperventilation: The Tip and the Iceberg', L. C. Lum, *Journal of Psychosomatic Research*, vol. 19, 1976.

'Hyperventilation and Cardiac Symptoms', P. G. F. Nixon, *Internal Medicine*, vol. 10, no. 12, 1989.

'The Hazards of Heavy Breathing', J. Perera, *New Scientist*, Dec. 1988

Two

What sort of people develop HVS?

All sorts, and at all ages.

Children are not exempt. Behavioural problems may be the first indication, and checking children's chests often reveals effortless, rapid upper-chest breathing, fuelling HVS symptoms.

Some women are sensitive to hormonal changes either during the week before their period, or in the latter stages of pregnancy. Higher progesterone levels increase the respiratory drive and may trigger HVS symptoms.

Women in labour often hyperventilate for long spells during rapid, painful contractions. In these circumstances prolonged over-breathing amplifies pain, making it more intense. Childbirth classes concentrate on breathing control and relaxation techniques to combat this.

People with asthma (15 per cent of New Zealand's population) are particularly prone to bad breathing habits and poor relaxation responses. Two or three decades ago physiotherapy was a top priority for people newly diagnosed with asthma. With the wonderful advances in user-friendly medications to control symptoms not many now benefit from learning breathing control, rest positions and relaxation — physical coping skills — to use while waiting for the asthma drugs to work.

This also applies to people with heart disease and hypertension. They may suffer chronic anxiety about their disorder, and poor breathing patterns increase their symptoms and heighten fears. While medications manage the disease, often little attention is paid to physical and emotional coping skills.

Older people having difficulties facing retirement and adjusting to ageing, loss or erratic health are prime candidates for HVS.

The condition is surprisingly common amongst teenagers, where pressures to conform (from parents), succeed (from teachers) and be cool (from friends) can be an unbearable burden.

High achievers seem to be in the firing line for developing HVS if they set their sights too high and fail to reach unrealistic aims.

Unfortunately, HVS is all too common in those who feel powerless, for whatever reason, and punish themselves for their perceived failures.

Sex, age and occupation are no barrier to HVS, as the following cases demonstrate. (Read through them again after you have finished the whole text.)

T, a 25-year-old woman, had recently moved to a new town and started a new high-pressure job where she was expected to be glamorous as well as clever. After a particularly bad few days when she felt she was not coping, she started to sleep poorly and felt increasingly anxious and irritable.

A former champion tennis player, T coached young players one evening a week, and found to her alarm her fitness levels had dropped drastically, with aching muscles and slowed reactions. Normally fit and energetic, she began to feel chronically tired and depressed. Her doctor prescribed sleeping pills to help break the insomnia/anxiety cycle, but by now her symptoms had escalated to shortness of breath for no apparent reason, often at rest, and occasional tingling lips and fingertips. For this her doctor prescribed a Ventolin inhaler, which was of no help. She periodically felt hot and clammy and was convinced she had a low-grade viral infection.

Her relationship with her boyfriend was becoming strained. She had completely lost interest in sex, and suspected that he thought she was being a hypo-chondriac.

Some months later, after a minor knee strain at tennis which needed treatment, T's physiotherapist noticed her frequent sighing and yawning and poor breathing pattern, and suggested an appointment with a respiratory physiotherapist. Her doctor supported this plan.

These signs were noted: her respiratory rate was 22

breaths a minute (the normal range is 10 to 14 breaths a minute) with a pulse rate of 90 beats a minute (average adult pulse rate is 72). She sighed eight times in two minutes (average adult sigh rate is once every five to 10 minutes).

While checking her breathing patterns, T had to loosen her tight-fitting belt before she could expand and breathe with her lower chest and diaphragm. She revealed that most of her clothes for work were tight fitting. (Hyperventilation Syndrome in the 1970s was also called the 'Designer Jeans Syndrome' — tight jeans restricted diaphragmatic breathing and shallow upper-chest rapid breathing became a habit.)

It took T several months to restore her breathing to a normal rate and pattern, with good days gradually starting to outnumber bad days as she put stress management techniques into action at work (along with elasticised waist-bands).

H, a 43-year-old secondary schoolteacher at a posh boys' school, had suffered mild asthma since childhood, but after a period of extra work at school he began experiencing anxiety attacks and bouts of shortness of breath for no particular reason. Thinking it was deteriorating asthma, he became depressed at his lack of physical fitness and coping abilities, and increased his asthma drugs.

When he was checked out by a chest physician, a hyperventilation component to his asthma symptoms was clearly seen. Even though H had previously been

taught to breathe well, he was amazed when
the physiotherapist pointed out his
upper-chest/mouth-breathing pattern.

Before a prone-lying relaxation session his
pulse rate was 96, his breathing rate was 22 per
minute, and his peak flow measurement (the
amount of air breathed out through a small
device people with asthma use to measure
wheeziness) was 480. After the session, his
breathing rate was 12, his pulse 80, and his peak
flow had improved to 620.

Over-breathing was making his asthma
symptoms worse, and the discovery of his ability
to help control tension and breathe correctly
was enough to motivate H to change his faulty
breathing pattern, practise regular relaxation
and improve his physical reserves with a
graduated walking programme.

O, a 54-year-old businessman, had suffered
a very mild stroke from which he had
completely recovered, but so anxious was he that it
would happen again, he became extremely tense
and depressed. Rapid breathing added real
symptoms to his imagined ones.

O became very isolated and felt he was letting his
family down. His wife had to drive him to his first
appointment with the physiotherapist. He was
restless, sighed three or four times a minute and
had cold clammy hands. His breathing rate was 20
per minute in an upper-chest/mouth-breathing
pattern. His pulse was 84.

He immediately grasped the concept
of over-breathing affecting blood-gas
levels and causing such widespread

symptoms, and after only two sessions was
breathing well, driving again and relieved of most
of his crippling anxieties.

A, 13 years old, terrified the staff at her school
as well as her parents with episodes of racing
heart rates, very rapid breathing (30 to 40 per
minute) and fainting. After a number of
trips by ambulance to Casualty, a respiratory
physician diagnosed Hyperventilation
Syndrome and mild asthma and referred her
to a respiratory physiotherapist for breathing
retraining, stress management and asthma
education. It turned out that A was having
problems adapting to her early blossoming
into a physically mature woman, well ahead
of her classmates.

· As is more common with teenage
hyperventilators, fainting was the most dramatic
symptom of A's habitual over-breathing. This
stopped almost immediately once she got over
the fear of the 'attacks', understood the rationale
behind them, and began using rest positions
and controlled breathing to cope with
sudden 'breathlessness'. She continued to
have outbreaks — before exams or during
times of conflict, but had the skills to deal
with the unpleasant symptoms at her command,
if she chose to.

P was a tall, glamorous, 43-year-old woman
who, two years ago, had given up a satisfying
part-time job because of 'poor health'. She had
suffered panic attacks while driving her car
and for about a year was unable to drive

down one particular stretch of road.

She was now a full-time housewife and mother, and did absolutely everything for her husband and three teenage sons. She had recently painted the whole exterior of the family house by herself, but brushed that off as 'nothing'. Her sense of self-worth was at ground level, and her family had adapted to her diminished estimation of herself as their slave. P was chronically tired and had completely lost the ability to tell the difference between normal tiredness and exhaustion. She only took to her bed if she had 'something wrong', which became increasingly common.

P's breathing rate at the first physiotherapy session was 25 per minute and her pulse rate was 90. She had attended antenatal classes for the births of her children, remembered diaphragmatic breathing and found it easy to do, but very hard to sustain. Relaxation was also extremely difficult and it was decided to leave exercise off her programme until diaphragmatic breathing was well established as a normal pattern and she had developed a good relaxation response.

A few days after the first session she telephoned to report that she felt worse than ever and that trying to relax was a major problem. At the next session it was decided to adopt a 'listening-relaxing' approach.

P loved music but had rarely listened to any in the past few years. She recorded the six Bach cello suites, each about 20 minutes long, on separate tapes and found listening to these while remaining still and totally relaxed a successful way to 'let go'. The music helped blot out the guilt she had previously felt when taking time out for herself to relax.

Low, slow breathing, rest and relaxation were top priorities for the first month. Her family were very helpful. P started a graduated walking programme in the fifth week, and after eight sessions at the clinic she felt she had the skills needed to continue on her own. A few months later she rang to say that she had driven down the stretch of road that had terrified her — a personal goal achieved.

J, a 44-year-old man running his own successful business, experienced episodes of chest pain and shortness of breath after a particularly busy spell. He was slightly overweight but exercised regularly and was reasonably fit. His GP referred him to a heart specialist, who found nothing wrong with J's heart. But he did notice J's erratic breathing and frequent sighs, and remarked on how restless and tense J was during the consultation. He was referred to a physiotherapy HVS clinic for assessment and management of his chronic HVS. He was fascinated with the physiological sequence of events due to over-breathing, which were causing him such trouble.

A habitual upper-chest breather, he found abdominal breathing hard to do.

A typical over-achiever, he decided after his first session to suppress his over-active upper chest the next day, by force, taping his chest from armpit to armpit with sticky tape! But by midday he was exhausted, his diaphragm not being strong enough to cope with the sudden change of pattern. (He was also very sore, after removing the tape.)

J made excellent progress, after deciding to take breathing retraining step by step, and establishing an effective relaxation response to counteract stress.

A , a superbly fit 26-year-old woman, visited her doctor because of episodes of breathlessness triggered by effort. Prior to this, running a marathon, she had been unable to finish because of chest discomfort. This had upset her, as she and her husband were soon planning a holiday which included running the New York marathon. Anxiety and upper-chest breathing became co-respondents in A's decline in energy and confidence. An extremely competitive person, A was very hard on herself for her perceived 'weakness'. After a visit to a respiratory physician, A was reassured that there was nothing wrong with her lungs, apart from mild hyperinflation of her chest (visible on X-ray). When she realised this was due to her chronic upper-chest/high volume breathing, she undertook breathing retraining. She reduced her breathing rate from 28 to 10 breaths a minute at rest, taking the pressure off her over-worked and often painful upper chest. Her running improved as she learned to restore 'low slow' breathing after effort. She completed the New York marathon.

Three

What is 'good breathing'?

Three groups of muscles are used for breathing:

The diaphragm
Tailor-made for each person to supply the right amount of air to the lungs during rest and normal activity, this strong, thin, flat sheet of muscle attached to the lower borders of the ribs separates the chest from the gut. Shaped rather like the dome of an umbrella, it flattens

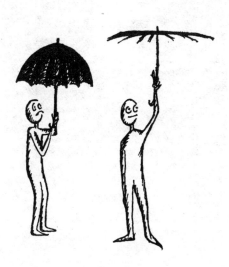

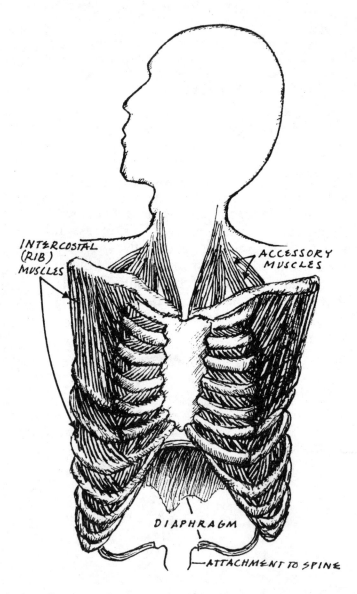

like a parasol to expand the lungs and draws in a sufficient air supply with very little effort.

The diaphragm acts as a vital pump, helping the heart circulate blood up and down the body. Diaphragmatic movement may vary from one centimetre at rest to 10 centimetres during vigorous activity.

Its gentle action also helps digestion.

Diaphragmatic breathing is the most energy-efficient and relaxing way to breathe.

Chest or intercostal muscles

These attach between each rib and tighten to lift the ribs, like birds' wings, expanding the chest wall to draw in air and contracting to push it out. They are used more during moderate-to-strong effort and use about 20 per cent more energy than the diaphragm.

Accessory muscles

These include shoulder and neck muscles used to tense the shoulders and lift the upper chest to help draw in extra air, and increase upper chest volumes. They can be seen working after strenuous exercise or effort. (In hyperventilators, they can be seen working in breathing rates of 20-breaths or more per minute.)

Abdominal muscles are also classed as accessory muscles.They can be felt working during moderate exercise, helping with breathing out.

In normal easy breathing 70 to 80% of the work of respiration is done by the diaphragm. The lower

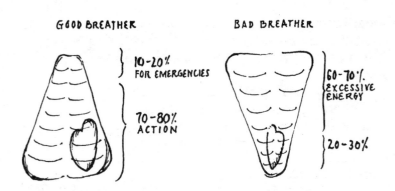

GOOD BREATHER

10-20% FOR EMERGENCIES

70-80% ACTION

BAD BREATHER

60-70% EXCESSIVE ENERGY

20-30%

chest or intercostal muscles do about 20 to 30 per cent of the work. The accessory muscles are used during and shortly after extremes in effort or stress. Habitual hyperventilators tend to reverse this ratio.

Oxygen and carbon dioxide levels, or blood gases, are kept in healthy balance by 12 regular breaths a minute (10 to 14 is an acceptable range) — moving about 600 cubic centimetres of air with each breath.

Nose-breathing is a major part of respiratory health. Air breathed in through the nose is:

• Warmed (lungs dislike cold, dry air).
• Moisturised (75 per cent humidification of inhaled air occurs in the nose and throat compared with 25 per cent via the mouth).
• Filtered (inhaled dust and debris are caught by tiny nasal hairs, not present in the mouth).

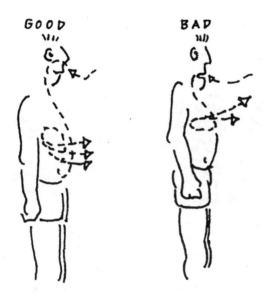

GOOD   BAD

The combination of cold, dry, unfiltered air being drawn in larger than normal quantities into the upper chest causes several problems in the respiratory system:

• Poor mixing and circulation of air throughout the lungs.
• Absorption and exchange of blood gases in the alveoli (air sacs) becomes less efficient.
• The body starts to suffer.

For people with persistent nasal problems who find it uncomfortable or too difficult to nose-breathe, and where nose drops, sprays and medications have stopped being effective, other treatment alternatives include:

• Physiotherapy. This offers non-invasive, painless

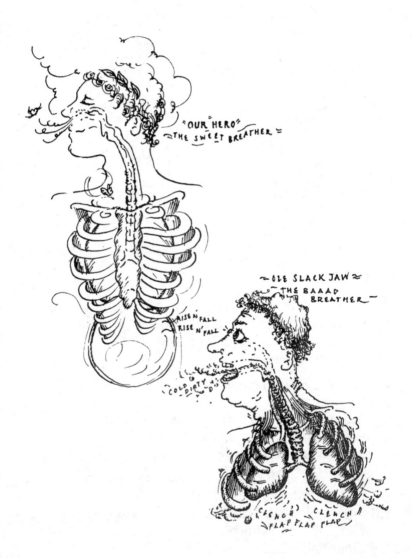

non-drug alternatives with short-wave or ultra-sound electrical treatments.

• Acupuncture. One study reported a 70 per cent success rate using this method to treat chronic rhinitis. The improvements lasted six or seven months, on average. If all else has failed, it is worth a try.

• Nasal washes. Stir a teaspoon of bicarbonate of soda and a teaspoon of salt into a glass of boiled water. When cool, pour into a clean, empty nasal spray bottle. Use as a 'wash' two or three times a day.

Why do people become hyperventilators?

The respiratory centre in the hind-brain responds to messages from different parts of the body as well as from the higher brain. After a bout of rapid breathing — whether from hard exercise, high emotions or danger — the respiratory system gradually allows the breathing rate to slow down as the body regains balanced blood gases. However, for some enduring prolonged stress, the respiratory centre slowly adapts to accept low or fluctuating carbon dioxide levels and respiratory alkalosis. So, while various parts of the mind and body may feel extremely unhappy about the blood-gas imbalance, the respiratory centre rides roughshod over any distress signals it receives, and keeps on instructing the lungs to breathe hard and fast.

The causes of this can be mechanical, starting after lung surgery or in lung diseases which cause air-flow disturbances (e.g., tuberculosis or bronchiectasis).

The problems may start after physical illnesses, such as chest infections, pneumonia, glandular fever or prolonged viral infections.

HVS often appears during or after emotional upheavals:

- Death of a partner/lover/family member;
- Separation and divorce;
- Losing a job or being made redundant;
- Changes of status/growing-up/ageing;
- Moving to a different town; or
- Living in a war zone.

Exercise, too, may trigger hyperventilation attacks where high stress levels and low physical reserves combine to bring on a sense of frustration, or even panic, as well as breathlessness.

What does it feel like to hyperventilate?

The most common phrases hyperventilators use are:

- 'I thought I was going to pass out — I couldn't seem to take the next breath in.'
- 'I never seem to be able to take a satisfying breath.'
- 'I've never felt quite the same since my operation/accident/break-up . . .'
- 'I really thought I was going crazy . . .'
- 'I thought I was dying . . .'

In sudden attacks, people are usually aware of their heaving upper-chest breathing and high anxiety, but are far more afraid of the strange symptoms that might follow, such as dizziness, tingling fingers and lips, and loss of concentration.

Those who go to their doctor may be prescribed a mild tranquilliser after a check-up and reassurance that 'nothing is wrong'. For some, this may be enough to break the cycle. But others who find their strange symptoms still lurking may start to imagine:

HEART ATTACK!
BRAIN TUMOUR!
BOWEL CANCER!

Do they go back to their doctor, or write their will?

Once the breathing pattern becomes centred in the upper chest and away from the diaphragm, more widespread and frightening symptoms begin to be felt.

The hazards of heavy breathing

• Habitual mouth-breathers develop irritable upper airways, with the risk of repeated throat infections. A very common sign of hyperventilation is repeated throat-clearing — the A-Hrrmm bug.
• Chronic hyperventilation triggers increased histamine levels in the blood. Sweaty palms and armpits, clammy skin and a flushed face are all signs of this. People with allergies such as hay fever, skin rashes, food intolerances or asthma find their symptoms are much worse.
• Response to pain is amplified, too, with stiffness,

aching and tension in muscles, tendons and joints, brought about by over-breathing, and poor metabolism, starting to feel like full-blown rheumatism.
• Heart disease-like symptoms, such as chest tightness or pain and palpitations, can be downright terrifying.
• Mental fuzziness, headaches or loss of concentration erodes self-confidence, especially if work suffers.
• Making love can become a nightmare — for both partners — if the 'heavy breathing' needed to achieve orgasm leads to a panic attack.
• Vivid dreams, nightmares and disturbed sleep patterns commonly accompany hyperventilation, making for round-the-clock distress.

The cycle is completed. Almost every system in the body suffers. Anxiety and fear of frightening symptoms drives the respiratory centre into top gear.

Hyperventilation Syndrome gives full throttle to the fear . . . and the symptoms . . . and bewilderment.

Further reading

'Acupuncture Therapy in Allergic Rhinitis', P. Chari, *American Journal of Acupuncture*, vol. 16, no. 2, 1988.
'Behavioural Breathlessness', J. B. L. Howell, *Thorax*, 45, 1990.
'Chronic Hyperventilation Syndrome', D. Innocenti in *Cash's Textbook of Chest, Heart and Vascular Disorders*, ed. P. A. Downie (4th edition, Faber and Faber, London, 1987).
'Dyspnoea: A Sensory Experience', R. Schwarztzstein *et al.*, *Lung*, vol. 168, 1990.
Respiratory Physiology, John B. West (4th edition, Williams and Wilkins, Baltimore, 1990).

Four

Is HVS very common?

British chest physician Claude Lum, who has done the most extensive documentation and clinical work on the subject over the last 30 years or so, has found that the problem is extremely widespread. About 12 per cent of any normal population are disordered breathers, and Lum maintains that numbers are increasing.

GPs generally agree that they would find 10 to 15 per cent of their patients to display signs of chronic hyperventilation. Specialists attract higher numbers, estimating that 50 to 70 per cent are habitual over-breathers. No figures are available from alternative health care sources.

Various studies from emergency coronary care unit admissions for chest pain have revealed that 30 to 40 per cent of the suspected heart attack victims had absolutely nothing wrong with their hearts.

How does a doctor know if symptoms are caused by HVS?

After a thorough check-up to rule out organic disease, the doctor may test for HVS by:

• The 12-Breath Test. The patient is asked to stand and take 12 rapid breaths, which many sufferers are amazed to find reproduces exactly their distressing symptoms.
• The Think Test. Breathing patterns are watched as the patient talks about symptoms and anxieties. Most people can pinpoint an event that caused them extreme stress which when they bring it to mind — along with their increased rate of breathing — also brings on most of their symptoms.

Other more high-tech methods of diagnosis are available, but because blood-gas levels fluctuate in chronic hyperventilators, it may be difficult to pick up the problem from a single test. Often patients have already been through batteries of stressful or painful tests, and many doctors prefer the direct 12-Breath or Think Tests to submitting their patient to more complex tests.

Unfortunately for those whose HVS symptoms include chest pain, it is one of the hardest to reproduce in the safety of the doctor's presence by over-breathing 'on command'.

There are three main types of chest pain associated with HVS:

• Sharp pains felt while breathing in — often just below the left breast — from pressure on the diaphragm by a bloated stomach, filled by 'air gulping', causing spasm of the diaphragm and pain.
• Dull aching pain with chest-wall soreness, most often felt after exercise. This is due to over-use of

chest-wall (intercostal) and accessory muscles, which tire easily and hurt.
• Heavy pain behind the breast bone radiating to the neck and arms. This happens when the blood supply to the heart muscle itself is reduced by HVS-stress-anxiety and spasming of coronary arteries.

In all three types of pain, many stresses (physical, social and emotional) may combine with hyperventilation to bring on chest pain — stresses not found in the security of the doctor's rooms.

What can be done for hyperventilators?

Unfortunately, many doctors fail to take account of the disabling effect of HVS and its habitual disordered breathing origins. Being told 'Go away, there's absolutely nothing wrong' may be briefly reassuring, but only until symptoms materialise again.

Often these seem infinitely worse. If no one believes the symptoms are real, does it mean that it's all in the mind? Or worse still, incurable. People who already have disorders such as asthma, heart disease or chronic pain which may be being made worse by erratic breathing are frequently loaded with extra drugs for the existing condition instead of being treated for the co-existing hyperventilation problem.

This is assuming that your doctor is even aware of HVS. High-tech medical training in recent years offers only passing mention of the subject — usually the acute phase — to trainee doctors. This results in doctors focusing only on symptoms, and in early pigeon-holing of their patients as suffering from 'anxiety neuroses', 'depression', or being 'panic-attack prone'. They then treat the symptoms of HVS, not the underlying over-breathing disorder (rather like prescribing skin lotion to someone with yellow jaundice).

Drug options

The most commonly prescribed drugs for these symptoms are tranquillisers, which act by burying the cause and leaves the over-breathing component untreated. While these may be life-savers in the short term, long-term use exposes patients to the added risks of dependency and addiction — and even further loss of self-confidence.

Courses of anti-depressants which are physically non-addictive are worth considering where disabling anxiety or phobias exist. They can be seen as an umbrella to shelter under, while restoring normal breathing patterns, learning physical coping skills and developing a confident relaxation response.

Physical coping skills

Long-term 'bad breathers' may need many physio-therapy sessions in breathing retraining and sorting out the often complex physical side effects that have radiated from HVS and its legacy of symptoms.

For instance, some chronic hyperventilators

develop avoidance behaviours in an attempt to control their symptoms. Chronic anxiety can lead to phobias — most commonly, fear of open spaces (agoraphobia) or enclosed spaces (claustrophobia). Common, too, is fear of travel; driving a car or fear of flying, for example.

Anxiety about sex can lead to loss of desire through fear of failure or fear of not being able to cope with intense emotions.

Expert help from a psychiatrist or psychologist would be indicated if these problems continued.

Where to start?

One doctor has described HVS as 'a diagnosis begging for recognition'. Once correctly diagnosed, the treatment is simple, although it requires commitment.

The six-step programme in the second part of this book uses the letters B E T T E R to cover important aspects of recovery:

- Breathing retraining.
- Exercise.
- Total body relaxation.
- Talk.
- Esteem.
- Rest and sleep.

The following six chapters outline one successful way to combat HVS and restore normal breathing patterns (and blood gases), and examine ways to help cope with the pressures that cause the problems.

Further reading

'Demonstration and Treatment of Hyperventilation Causing Asthma', G. Hibbert and D. Pilsburn, *British Journal of Psychiatry*, vol. 153, 1988.

'Hypertension and Hyperventilation — a common combination that is rarely diagnosed', Norman M. Kaplan, *Cardiology Guide*, October 1989.

'Psychogenic Breathlessness and Hyperventilation', L. C. Lum, *Update*, May 1987.

'Respiratory and psychiatric abnormalities in chronic symptomatic hyperventilation', C. Bass and W. N. Gardner, *British Medical Journal*, vol. 290, 1985.

Five

Breathing retraining

Nobody needs to be shown how to breathe, but many people are disorganised breathers, using their upper-chest muscles instead of their diaphragms.

For people with HVS, restoring a normal breathing pattern may take time and a lot of regular practice. Some are able to switch easily to low, slow, diaphragm breathing, while others may take months, sometimes up to a year, to change their ways. The following simple techniques will help turn you into a good breather, but if you continue to have problems seek extra help from a respiratory physiotherapist.

The four basic steps to follow are:

- Becoming aware of faulty breathing patterns.
- Learning to nose-diaphragm breathe.
- Suppressing upper-chest movement during normal breathing.
- Reducing breathing to a slow, even, rhythmic rate — the average breathing rate for adults is about 12 breaths per minute; two to three seconds breathe in; three to four seconds out.

Big versus deep breaths

People learn from a very early age, often at school, to stick out their chests and hold in their stomachs like soldiers or beauty queens when asked to breathe. Ask anyone to take a *deep* breath and chances are that they will puff up their upper chest and take a *big* breath instead.

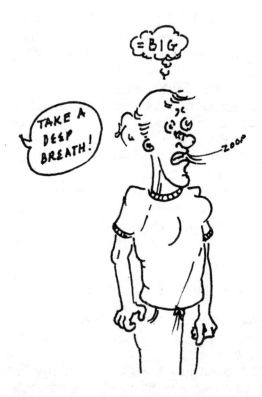

Try it. First, place the hand you write with on your stomach between your lower ribs and navel. Put the other hand on your breastbone, just below your collar-

THE LUNG~HO SALUTE

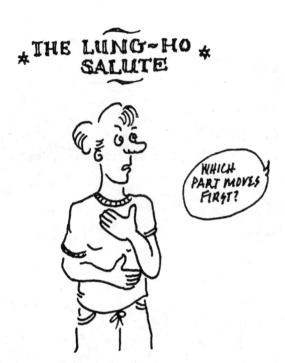

bones (the Lung Ho salute, with apologies to Rewi Alley).

Take a *deep* breath and notice:

- Which part of your chest moved first?
- Which part of your chest moved most?
- Did you breathe in through your mouth or nose?

If you breathed in through your nose, your stomach expanded first and you felt almost no upper-chest movement, you are breathing in a natural pattern.

If you breathed in fast through your mouth, your upper chest heaved first and you felt little or no

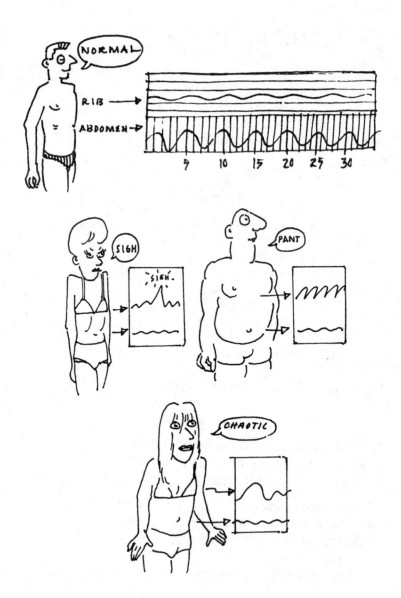

movement under your writing hand, or
your stomach drew in, you are a disordered
breather.

Strategies for breathing retraining

Practise lying comfortably on your back, head
well supported with pillows or cushions. Let as
much air as possible sigh out of your lungs
without pushing. Shoulder and upper-chest
relaxation is vital here.

With lips together, jaw relaxed, draw air
slowly in through your nose, relaxing and
expanding your waist so your stomach puffs
up. Let the air 'fall' out of your chest — also
through the nose — as the elastic recoil of your
lower chest and diaphragm breathes air out
effortlessly.

*Take very small abdominal breaths at first, making
sure you start each in breath with the diaphragm, and let
go at the end of the breath out.*

Mentally repeat to yourself: 'Lips together, jaw
relaxed, breathing low and slow.'

Imagine a fine piece of elastic round your waist,
stretching as you inhale; or think of breathing into
your belt or waist-band. Check chest movement
using the Lung Ho salute.

Timing

Once you feel confident about the breathing
pattern, concentrate on the rate. Have a
watch or clock with a second hand easily
visible. Watch the second hand for half a minute
while you count your breaths. (Breathing

in and out counts as one breath.)

Aim to reduce your breathing rate to 12 breaths a minute — six per half minute. If you are much faster than that — relax — let go — and check the clock again in a couple of minutes.

Focus on the evenness, gradually increasing the time taken to breathe in and out. Breathing out usually takes slightly longer than breathing in, with a relaxed pause at the end of exhalation. This may be more pronounced in people with chest disorders such as asthma or chronic airway limitation (CAL).

Practise the new low, slow breathing pattern lying on your side, sitting and standing. As you get better at it try breathing this way while walking.

At first, if you have been addicted to mouth/upper-chest breathing, nose/diaphragm breathing will feel very peculiar. Some people describe it as 'back to front' breathing. Others report uncomfortable feelings of 'air hunger'. This is a good sign as it shows your respiratory centre is being challenged to accept normal CO_2 levels.

It can take a long time and constant practice to get

When you feel breathless

Stop
Drop (your shoulders and upper chest),
Flop (relax).
Use the rest positions illustrated overleaf when and wherever you become short of breath and need to focus on low, slow breathing.

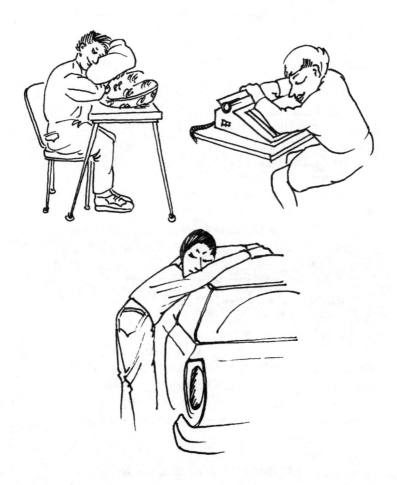

your diaphragm strong and working confidently
— and for your respiratory centre to accept
normal blood gas levels. Don't be hard on
yourself if you slip back to erratic breathing
habits. Just concentrate on the next breath and
getting it right.

How often?

Before you get out of bed every morning, lie
on your back for a few minutes practising
relaxed low, slow breathing, to establish the
pattern for the day.

During the day, check with the Lung Ho salute,
every hour on the hour.

Check your breathing pattern — correct it —
then FORGET IT.

Constant repetition is the best way to reinforce
your healthy breathing pattern. But don't be
obsessive.

In bed at night, repeat the morning
breathing routine lying on your side to
help you get to sleep.

As you become accustomed to breathing
this way, the need to Lung Ho will be less,
as you develop better breathing awareness.
During stressful times though, it pays to
check your breathing pattern and rate.
Concentrating on something physical helps
dampen anxieties.

Common mistakes and problems

Your diaphragm may be jumpy at first, especially if
it has been out of action for a long time.

- Like any other group of muscles which have been

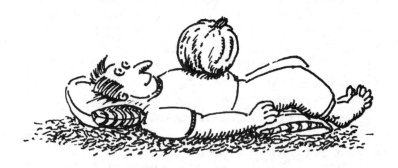

out of use, the diaphragm itself may need strengthening. If you find yourself breathing in a jerky, 'staircase' fashion, mildly resisted breathing with a two-kilogram bag of rice or sugar (one woman found her iron made a perfect weight) on your stomach helps focus on the right pattern. Place the weight just below your navel, lying on your back, and practise for ten minutes twice a day for a week.

If you have problems with gastric reflux (heartburn), practise in a semi-reclining position.

• People on courses of steroid tablets, such as Prednisone, need to pay special attention to maintaining diaphragm strength. Loss of condition, in big muscle groups (thigh muscles for example) is a common side effect. The diaphragm is not exempt. Strengthening exercises restore muscle power.

• Those with asthma — children and adults — also need to pay special attention to their breathing after a bout of wheezing. Breathing may be chaotic during an attack, switching from upper-chest to diaphragmatic, with little chance of control; this is normal as an increased respiratory drive is natural at this time. But using rest positions and the 'Stop, Drop, Flop' routine helps combat the fear and anxiety while waiting for the asthma medications to work. Once the attack is over, re-establishing a low, slow nose-breathing pattern and suppressing upper-chest use must be top priority.

• Your body will play all sorts of tricks to start you over-breathing again. The urge to sigh, yawn or 'air-gulp' and race back to hyperventilation will seem overwhelming at times, and very uncomfortable at first. Remember, this is a good sign, showing you are making progress.

Remind yourself that your respiratory centre is frantically trying to make you hyperventilate again. But with regular and determined practice your respiratory centre will readjust to accept a balanced pH and normal ventilation. To help resist the urge to take a big breath in try swallowing hard, and continue breathing low and slow.

• Another common trick is to 'brace' or fill up the upper chest, holding in huge volumes of air while using the diaphragm to breathe in more. Breathing this way will make symptoms worse.

It is equally important to suppress high, upper-chest breathing and relax shoulders and chest as it is to centre breathing low and slow.

An excellent image to use in focusing on low, slow breathing is to imagine breathing through your heels.

When you feel your breathing going high (with sighs) remember to:

- Relax your shoulders by using a rest position.
- Keep lips together, jaw relaxed, shoulders down.
- Concentrate totally on low, slow breathing until you start to feel in, not out of, control.

In other words . . . 'Stop, Drop, Flop'.

Further reading

The Body in Question, Jonathan Miller (Jonathan Cape, London, 1978).

'CO_2 Response and Pattern of Breathing in Patients with Symptomatic Hyperventilation, Compared to Asthmatic and Normal Subjects', J. Hormbrey *et al., European Respiratory Journal* 1, 1988.

'Handling the Chronic Hyperventilation Patient', A. Pilgrim, *Physiotherapy*, vol. 72, no. 6, 1986.

'Physiotherapy in Respiratory Care', A. Hough (Chapman and Hall 1992) pgs 129-134.

Physiotherapy Management of Chronic Hyperventilation, I. Rowbottom, ACPRC *Journal* No. 21, 1992.

Six

Esteem

Most habitual hyperventilators suffer from a battered self-image, one of the first major casualties in an outbreak of HVS. Good days may be few and far between, and these are overshadowed by fear and loathing of bad days. Gradual erosion of confidence — feeling that you are letting people down — also adds to a general sense of lack of self-worth. Strong positive emotions such as love, happiness and laughter gradually get pushed aside by anger (often repressed), anxiety and depression.

Most people get a lot of attention during times of major upheaval. Little attention, though, is paid to the cumulative effects of minor, everyday niggles. Often left unresolved, these can build up to major proportions if allowed. Learning to say 'sorry but no' to demands you know will overload you is a very important skill to master.

The power of laughter

Loosening up, relaxing and finding some humour in your life will prove that laughter, as well as being the best medicine, is also a powerful and non-toxic remedy. Laughter benefits the whole person, body and soul. A good laugh liberates minds from repetitive, often negative thought patterns. The body's immune system is boosted, too. One humour researcher found increased levels of immunoglobulins (antibodies) were produced in people watching funny films over those watching dull documentaries. Laughter also seems to reduce output of the stress hormone adrenalin; and just as exercise releases opio-peptides (hormones that make you feel good) so does laughter. The final bonus is the immediate and exquisite relaxation that follows laughter.

Use of language

Breaking the tension ' HVS ' anxiety ' HVS cycle needs a firm commitment to changing your outlook as well as your breathing patterns. Language and choice of words play an important part here. To start, cross the words 'should', 'if only' and 'what if' out of your vocabulary.

Awareness of thought and speech patterns — with fragmented, illogical and mostly negative phrases dominating — can be changed. If you catch yourself thinking things like 'I'll never be able to manage', or 'I'm always letting people down', gently question yourself — never? or always? — and *think* about it. Break the line of despair.

Depression

Fear of losing control is especially strong in chronic hyperventilators. This often leads to repression of normal emotions, and the withholding of love, warmth, anger or sadness. Unexpressed grief, fear or resentment puts people in the fast lane to depression and withdrawal from everyday life.

At the risk of giving depression a good name, it is a fairly normal reaction to prolonged bouts of hyperventilation and the resulting nasty symptoms. If there is nothing concrete to 'cut out' or take a pill for, anxiety and depression are reasonable enough reactions to feeling constantly off-centre. Being diagnosed as

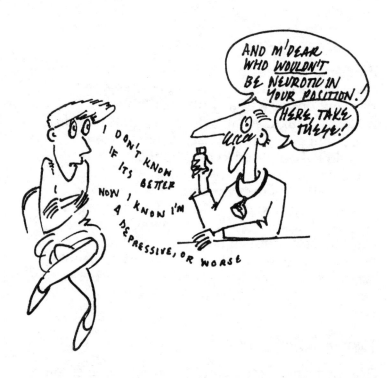

suffering from anxiety and depression is undermining enough. Unfortunately, treating the symptoms of these without first sorting out the basic breathing disorder is going to be of limited value to the individual, and of great expense to our health-care system. Chemical happiness in the form of prescribed tranquillisers or recreational drugs must be approached with extreme caution and full information.

More sinister though, with the accompanying wearing away of self-esteem, is the likelihood of turning hyperventilators into chronic invalids. Being shunted from specialist to specialist trying to find a diagnosis — undergoing all sorts of sometimes risky investigations or drug therapies with no relief — is it surprising that anxiety and depression become chronic?

Failure to recognise over-breathing, and exhaustion, denial of normal tiredness, and abusing stimulants, such as coffee and cigarettes (and worse) to boost flagging energy levels, is asking for trouble once your nervous system starts signalling distress. Many people — mature, intelligent, even clever people — are positively backward at recognising signs of exhaustion. These can include:

- Increased heart and breathing rate.
- Mental and physical restlessness and difficulty relaxing.
- Slowed reactions and reflexes.
- Inability to concentrate.
- Irritability, and a tendency to fly off the handle.

- Loss of energy and stamina.
- Poor resistance to colds and flu.
- Loss of interest in sex.

Someone with a healthy self-image is much more likely to take notice of their body's reactions to tiredness, stress and the early signs of exhaustion. Developing a sense of balance between effort (good for the ego), relaxation (physical and mental rejuvenation), sleep (recovery), and exercise (increasing physical reserves) is a good way to rebuild esteem of yourself and others.

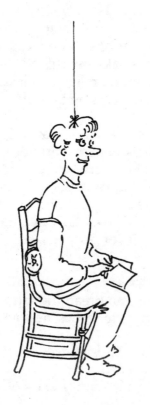

Body mechanics and posture

Good posture, too, is a very important ingredient in strengthening self-confidence. Check regularly: imagine being suspended by a fine thread from the back of the top of your head; stretch up tall to prevent the phantom thread breaking.

Always sit with your bottom snug against the back of the chair. Maintaining a lumbar hollow when sitting stops your upper spine from sagging and compressing your chest.

Apart from the mechanical advantages to the process of breathing itself, holding and carrying yourself well — standing or sitting — makes you feel in charge and physically confident.

Tell a friend

Another potent way of taking the fear out of HVS and giving yourself power over it is to undertake to tell five people you know about it. Explain the syndrome, its effects, and how you handle it. Unravelling the tight spiral of HVS can be a long, yet illuminating process. Gaining insight into the mechanisms that bring on HVS symptoms is only the starting point though.

Once you have grasped this point, plenty of help is available out in the community to help rebuild a healthy self-image, if you need it. Family, individual and group counselling is available from a variety of agencies. Check out your local library for information, and browse through the dozens of excellent self-help books on the shelves. Coming to grips with HVS, and getting it off your chest will put you back in the driving seat and in, not under — or out of — control.

Further reading

'Exhaustion: Cardiac Rehabilitation's Starting Point', P. G. F. Nixon, *Physiotherapy Journal*, May 1986.
Feel the Fear and Do It Anyway, Susan Jeffers (Century, London, 1989).

Seven

Total body relaxation

Hyperventilators, who may have been struggling for months, even years, with over-breathing, bizarre symptoms, fear and tension, find it extremely hard to let go and relax. Releasing physical tension helps let go mental stress — the rats-in-the-brain repetitive thoughts that go round and round in the mind. This negative internal chatter-box can be just as hard to subdue as trigger-happy lungs.

Learning the knack of switching on relaxation if familiar HVS symptoms reappear — and they will in times of stress — is an effective way of stopping symptoms in their tracks. It may be difficult at first to feel confident that you can release tension, and to take time for yourself to practise relaxation techniques. But daily relaxation does help unknot your life. It gives you more reserves to cope with daily stresses — good and bad — which are part of normal life.

All relaxation techniques start with low, slow diaphragmatic breathing, so mastering Chapter 5 is essential before continuing further with learning total body relaxation.

Choosing a suitable relaxation method

There are several methods to choose from. Your choice will depend on whether mental or physical tension is more of a problem, and where you are at the time. Knowing different methods makes you more adaptable. Most public hospital physiotherapy outpatient departments teach various types of relaxation as part of general stress management.

To get started, try the *Hyperventilator's Special* or *Prone Lying Relaxation* (lying on your front).

This method specially suits people who at first feel vulnerable or ill at ease trying to learn to relax lying on their backs. Lying face down has a built-in sense of safety, with the soft 'under-belly' protected by the 'tough shell', or spine.

The main elements of relaxation can be practised. These include:

- Diaphragmatic breathing.
- Switching off antigravity or posture reflexes.
- Arousing awareness of tension areas in the body.
- Reducing entropy of the body. (Entropy is the measurement of energy or heat generated in the body not used for work. Think of a tense person perched on the edge of a chair, using ten times more energy than necessary to keep upright.)

Learning to recognise 'stress zones' in various groups of muscles helps heighten awareness of the powerful switch conscious relaxation can be.

Preparation
- Set aside a time — at least 10 to 15 minutes.
- Choose a quiet place in which to practise.
- Take the telephone off the hook, or turn down the bell volume.
- Tell people around you what you are going to do and why, and ask them not to disturb you for that time. Even quite young children can learn to be co-operative about 'your time'. Some may even enjoy being time-keeper.

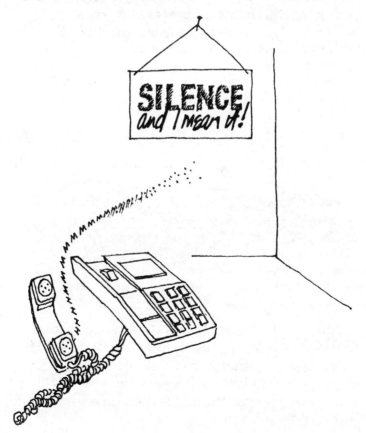

- Schedule regular times for practice instead of 'finding' time. If you keep a diary, mark time out for relaxation breaks.

Technique
Lying face down on a firm bed or on the floor, place a rolled blanket or firm pillow under your hips (to free the diaphragm) and under your ankles. You may need a soft pillow under your upper chest if you have a stiff neck.

If you can lie with your arms up, hands under your head, this helps suppress upper-chest breathing (like the forward-leaning rest position). If your shoulders are uncomfortable, keep arms by your sides.

Don't go to sleep in this position if you have restricted neck movement.

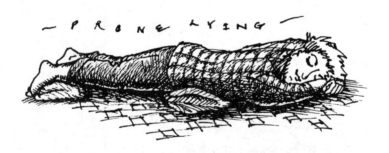

You can practise some of the mental relaxation techniques (below) or listen to soothing music. After an initial concentration on breathing low and slow for three or four breaths, forget about your chest and . . . let go. Relaxing in this position is surprisingly rejuvenating.

Progressive Physical Relaxation

This involves methodically stretching big groups
of muscles for five to six seconds and letting go
for 15 to 20 seconds, concentrating on feeling
the difference between tension and release. This
is an excellent way of pinpointing tension
zones, such as neck, scalp, shoulders, hands
and lower back. The majority of people taken
through Progressive Physical Relaxation are
extremely surprised at the amount of physical
strain they have been holding on to, and
are even more surprised at how good it feels to
let it go.

Technique

Lying on your back on a bed or the floor, cover up
with a blanket, with a pillow under your head and
knees.

Start with two or three low, slow breaths, then
forget your breathing while you gently tighten the
muscles of your left ankle — pulling your toes up
towards you and pressing your left knee into the
pillow, tightening your whole leg to the hip. (Your
left heel will lift off the bed.) Hold for five seconds
— and let go slowly, and relax for 15 to 20 seconds.
Repeat with the right leg.

Continue with the same timing as you go on to
stretch and elongate the fingers and thumb of your
left hand. Let go slowly and . . . relax. Repeat with
the right hand.

Push your left elbow gently into the bed. Let
go slowly and . . . relax. Repeat with your right
elbow.

71

Slide both your hands down the bed or floor towards your feet, feeling the stretch to the shoulders and neck muscles. Let go slowly and . . . relax.

Tuck in your chin and gently press your head back into the pillow, being aware of stretching the long muscles up the back of your neck. Let go slowly and . . . relax.

Very lightly, bring your teeth together. With lips remaining closed, separate your teeth a little and push your lower jaw forward . . . and relax, and swallow . . . being aware of your tongue resting on the floor of your mouth, not clenched up against the roof.

Screw up your nose . . . and let go and . . . relax.

Think of your eyelids as light as feathers, resting softly over your eyes. With eyes remaining closed, raise your eyebrows as high as you can . . . and let go slowly . . . feeling your brow and scalp smooth and relaxed. This is often a tense area. Repeat two or three times.

Imagine all tension leaving your body through the top of your head.

Check 'tension zones', and repeat sequences in those areas that still feel tight. You may have to repeat tensing/relaxing routines 10 or more times in some stress areas before you feel release.

When you feel you have unwound physically, rest and enjoy the feeling. Keep nagging or disruptive thoughts out of your mind by focusing on neutral repetitive ones — mentally chanting your two-times tables, for example.

The whole process at first usually takes 10 to 15 minutes. When it is time to stop (checking your watch will not disturb relaxation), take two or three low, slow breaths and have a good stretch before slowly getting up.

Adapting this method to practise sitting upright in a chair is easy, and can be used at work or on planes, buses, or trains.

To learn the sequences, it may help to ask someone to read out the orders for you, or to tape yourself reading the sequences — with timing — to play back to yourself, perhaps with soothing music to follow. Music for Airports by Brian Eno is an excellent example of 'switching off' music, with its slow, rhythmic, ethereal sounds.

Mental relaxation techniques

The most popular methods are:

Passive Mental Relaxation
This involves sitting comfortably, eyes closed, hands on thighs, palms of the hands turned up, and after the first three or four low, slow breaths, not thinking about breathing or trying to relax but passively accepting

whatever floats through the mind. Concentration is focused by silent repetition of sounds. (For example, repeat the word 'one' with each breath out.) Along with mental relaxation, a deep physical relaxation is experienced as well.

Transcendental Meditation (TM)
Based on the above technique, an individual word is given, to be repeated silently and rapidly, focusing on deep physical and mental relaxation. Nagging conscious thoughts are pushed out by the silent repetition of your word. Most major towns have a TM centre. Introduced to the West nearly 30 years ago, it has remained a popular relaxation/meditation method. Although it is relatively expensive, people who have difficulty getting started with relaxation may enjoy the group support.

Auto Hypnosis
This mental relaxation method involves sitting fully supported in a chair about three metres from a wall, focusing on a spot slightly above eye level. Counting breaths back from 100, picture yourself 'floating' and 'free'. As your eyes start to feel heavy, let them close, and stop counting when you feel floppy and pleasantly relaxed.

You will be fully awake and aware of your surroundings and able to check your watch, to time your relaxation. When you want to finish, count three breaths to slowly revert to 'normal', while holding on to the pleasant relaxed feeling.

Creative Visualisation

Setting yourself up as for other methods (sitting, or lying on your back or stomach), creative visualisation involves relaxing around positive and pleasurable mental images. By mentally involving all your senses — imagining tastes, smells, textures and sounds — you build up a rich picture in your mind. Remembering, for example, a childhood picnic, reliving the sounds of the sea, hot sun on your skin (without having to worry about sunscreen!), sand between your toes, the smell and textures of peeling an orange, and the sweet taste of its flesh, can be physically and mentally relaxing.

Taking time to build up a rich, complex, pleasurable picture can also include creative visualisations of positive actions taken by you to release tension, such as imagining slowly and methodically unknotting a rope bound around your problems.

About two billion brain cells make up our speech and conscious thought centres. But our unconscious is

Body systems	During relaxation	Under stress
Breathing rate	Down	Up
Heart rate	Down	Up
Blood pressure	Down	Up
Blood supply to muscles and organs	Up	Down
Muscle tension	Down	Up
Adrenalin output	Down	Up, up, up,

made up of 100 billion brain cells, and our visual sense operates mainly in this larger area. No one has worked out why, but our brains do not differentiate between vividly imagined events and real ones. When you think about a painful or frightening situation, your body reacts as though it was really happening (as in the Think Test). Recent experiments on the muscles of people with back pain show that muscle tension increased between two and six times when the person being tested simply thought about their pain. Reversing this response makes sense. Relaxation with visualisation is a very potent natural relaxant.

Other methods of relaxation

• Joining a yoga class is an excellent way of combining exercise, breathing and relaxation all in one. Most classes finish with a 20-30 minute total body and mind relaxation session. Some classes teach meditation techniques for home practice as well. Joining a class is often the best way for busy people to schedule, without guilt, time for themselves. Avoid the more advanced breathing exercises at first. (Practise your own 'low, slow' pattern.) Shop around and find a class that suits you.

• Treating yourself to a regular back or full body massage from a reputable masseur is an excellent alternative to the more cerebral approaches to relaxation. People who have been long-time hyperventilators frequently have stiff, tense upper spines and knotty muscles with painful trigger points. Having these gently kneaded and loosened up can make you feel as though you have had three relaxation sessions and a good night's sleep rolled into one.

• Practise gentle stretches of tense muscle groups.

• Having a facial is another way of taking time out; both men and women report it to be intensely relaxing.

• Dubbed by one wit as 'wooden Valium', rocking back and forth in a rocking chair is a tried and true method of relaxing, from infancy through to old age. Many people recovering from HVS swear by this as a 'quick-fix' relaxation method.

How often — how long?

Feeling good enough about yourself to make regular relaxation a priority is important, because regular practice is essential. To start with, you may not feel much immediate benefit; it is often other people who remark on changes and improvements.

The ideal is to weave two 10-15 minute-long relaxation sessions into your day. Experiment with different methods for different times of the day and week. Sometimes, in the early days, unpleasant reactions to 'letting go' puts hyperventilators off continuing with relaxation, but it is worth persevering. HVS feeds on tension and anxiety. Try another method.

Regular practice increases your general awareness of stresses and strains and the need to let go shoulders and upper chest muscles.

Once you develop an effective relaxation response 'mini-relaxes' practised several times during the day may be sufficient — checking and releasing tension zones at the same time as you check your breathing pattern with the Lung Ho salute.

Just as you recognise triggers that bring on hyperventilation, create some relaxation triggers of your own to combat it. Small things such as mentally repeating the phrase 'Lips together, jaw relaxed, breathing low and slow', turning your palms up and letting your shoulders relax, or pressing stress-releasing trigger points in the muscles on the backs of your hands between the thumb and index finger help switch off tension.

Remind yourself how much energy you are wasting by being physically tense. Physical tension goes hand in hand with the negative mental chatterbox that constantly undermines your feelings of well-being.

Remind yourself that relaxation only helps eliminate the symptoms, not the causes of stress.

Develop the ability to 'accept the things you cannot change — have the courage to change the things you can, and the wisdom to know the difference' (to borrow from the Alcoholics Anonymous prayer). Addiction to bad breathing can be a hard habit to break.

Check your shoulders, elbows and hands when walking, and make sure they are not tight and clenched. If they are, it means you are carrying your stress with you, like heavy unwanted baggage.

Look in your local library for books and tapes on relaxation.

Make regular total body relaxation as important, and regular, as cleaning your teeth.

Further reading

The Relaxation Response, Herbert Benson (Fount Paperbacks, London, 1977).

Simple Relaxation, Laura Mitchell (John Murray, London, 1988).

Super Health, booklet and tape, available from Mental Health Foundation branches.

Visualisation for Change, Patrick Fanning (New Harbinger Press, Oakland, 1988).

Eight

Talk

Talking can be a major problem for over-breathers for two reasons. The first is breath control while speaking. (And the one thing you really need to be able to do, through the power of speech, is to express ideas and emotions — to your doctor and to people close to you.) Using quick, gasping upper-chest mouth breaths while talking can trigger HVS symptoms. Slightly husky, light speech, punctuated by throat clearing, sniffing, sighing or yawning often indicates hyperventilation.

Marilyn Monroe's sexy breathless voice may have had more to do with an overactive upper chest, her waist pinioned by a cinch belt, than true desire! A full-toned confident voice needs good breath control: ask any politician, actor, or singer.

Tips for breath control while speaking:

• Relax your shoulders and low, slow nose-breathe before speaking.
• Draw air in through your nose between sentences while talking instead of quickly gulping in air through your mouth.
• Mentally put commas and pauses into your speech.

- Practise speaking in front of a mirror. Recite the alphabet or two-times table. Use the Lung Ho salute to check chest movement.
- Remember to swallow and relax your shoulders if you get an irresistible urge to yawn, sigh or take a big breath.
- Watch other people's breathing patterns when they speak. Listen during telephone conversations. See if you can spot another hyperventilator.
- Always be aware of centering your breathing — low and slow.
- Combining eating and talking with breath control is a big problem for some. Most of the best advice about relaxed eating was taught to us as infants by our parents:

> Always sit down to eat. *Never eat on the run.*
> Avoid talking with your mouth full.
> Nose-breathe while chewing.
> Eat slowly.
> Eat very small mouthfuls.
> Chew thoroughly.
> Never eat slumped in a low chair.
> Drink slowly too, holding your breath as you sip, to prevent air-gulping. (Drinking through a straw may be helpful.)

If breath control while speaking or eating continues to be a problem, seek expert advice from a speech therapist.

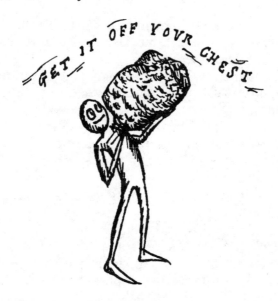

The second area where talking may be difficult is fear of voicing deep anxieties about HVS symptoms. Bottling up problems is not good for your health. Anxiety increases mental and physical tension and adrenalin output, revving up the heart and breathing rates, and HVS. Recent research has scientifically proved that thinking or talking about physical symptoms can both directly and indirectly affect the body's physiology — a fact known unscientifically since the dawn of time. (An example of the direct effect of thought on physiology is, of course, the Think Test.)

Repression / depression

The indirect physiological effect lies in the relationship between stress and depression. Experiencing loss of control over parts of your life (as felt with HVS) is a major ingredient in depression. A sense of isolation develops if you are afraid of confiding in anyone. (Worse still if you do, and are disbelieved or thought neurotic.) Lacking confidence to cope socially or keep up friendships, or thinking you are letting family, friends or work-mates down is a common sign of anxiety and a potent depressant.

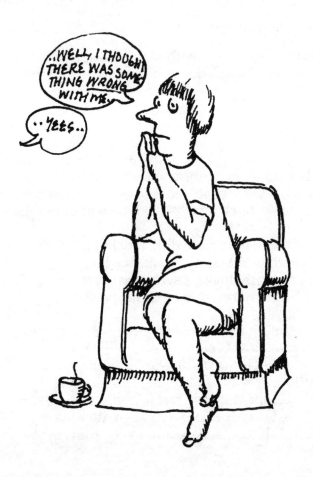

Can you hear me?

Listening skills often need brushing up, too.
Expression and communication are very much
two-way processes. People close to you may have
become alarmed, confused or even bored by your
real and imagined disorders. Relaxing enough to be
able to listen to other people is as necessary as
finding someone who will listen to you.

Deciding to change

Scientific medicine, with high-tech surgical and
pharmaceutical interventions, has revolutionised
the 'healing arts' over the last 20 years. But it
has also produced a society that holds an
unrealistic belief in drugs as the cure-all, which has
instilled a passive attitude to becoming well.
Recovery from HVS requires an active involvement
and personal commitment. And talking — being
able to identify problems and confront the need for
acceptance or change — is a vital part of reducing
stress.

For those who have difficulty identifying
the sources of anxiety, sessions with a
clinical psychologist, psychiatrist or therapist
may be of enormous benefit in speeding up
recovery.

Regaining a resonant confident voice comes
with low, slow breathing, relaxation and talking
out and releasing bottled-up resentments and
emotions.

Find someone you trust to confide in. Use
positive language, and, starting with the next
breath, talk yourself up and away from HVS.

Further reading

Listen to Me, Listen to You, Anne Kotzman (Penguin Books, Melbourne, 1989).

Mental Health for Women, Hilary Haines (Reed Methuen, Auckland, 1985).

Will the Real Mr New Zealand Please Stand Up?, Gwendoline Smith (Penguin Books, Auckland, 1990).

Nine

Exercise

Hyperventilation Syndrome and low
physical fitness tend to go hand in hand.
The effects of inactivity — sluggish circulation,
achey muscles, lack of energy and shortness
of breath — all add to a general loss of self-
confidence.

This is most often due to:

• Fear of triggering uncontrollable rapid breathing
during effort.
• Panic about not being able to draw the next
breath in.
• The side-effects of poor sleep and depression.
• Fear of fatigue.

Nearly all chronic hyperventilators complain of
muscle fatigue. The most common types
complained of are central fatigue, with
generalised feelings of low energy; and
peripheral fatigue, felt in the limbs, where
muscles tire easily and protest.

Why is physical fitness important in HVS?

Physical fitness is described in the 'Teachers'
Guide for Fitness for Living' (*Clinical
Management*, vol. 9, no. 3) as 'the body's

ability to meet the normal demands of everyday life — work and recreation — with ease, and with enough margin to adequately cope with emergencies'. Most hyper-ventilators would admit falling far behind this description.

Everybody feels better when they have reserves of energy to spare. Feeling fit has added bonuses. It leads to improvement of body image and a stronger sense of self-reliance. Enjoyment of regular physical exercise and the sense of confidence it brings is a vital part of banishing HVS.

Does it have to be vigorous?

The three main ingredients in improving physical fitness are:

• Endurance exercise. This trains the body to 'work' for long periods of time, by improving heart and circulation (cardio-vascular) fitness (e.g., running, jogging or aerobics classes).
• Strengthening exercise. Specific groups of muscles are trained to improve function and prevent injury during particular leisure or work-related effort (e.g., leg-muscle strengthening for skiers).
• Flexibility exercise. Joints and muscles are kept supple and able to move through a full range of movement, to prevent muscle imbalances that might lead to injury or, in the long term, osteoarthritis (e.g., dance, stretch or yoga classes, and swimming).

While all three ingredients are important in a balanced fitness programme, emphasis in recent times has leaned towards the cardiovascular. The fitness boom of the last decade has given the impression that to become fit means being encased in bri-nylon and working out in gyms. Many people torture their bodies into fitness levels way beyond their needs, but the byproduct of this — feeling healthy and on top of the world — keeps them at it.

Be realistic

The risk of injury in these endurance-based, high-impact pastimes is high, especially if previously unfit people take them on without preparation. During high-impact exercise, such as aerobics and running, the feet hit the ground with a force between two and four times the body weight. You need to be *basically* fit even to start these, in order to avoid strains, sprains and pain.

Low-impact exercise options — brisk walking, cycling, low-resistance circuit training (if you want to join a gym) and swimming — are great ways to improve fitness for the average person's needs. There are plenty of other ways — enjoying gardening, playing outdoor games with your kids, going dancing or walking the dog are all excellent 'body boosters'.

Getting started

People who suffer from hyperventilation tend to be over-achievers. Make sure progress is gradual. Take it easy. Include a friend or

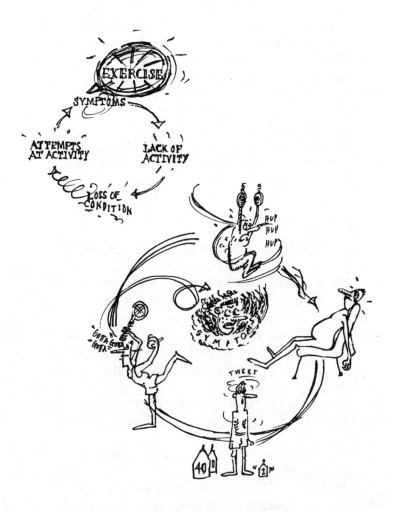

partner who knows about your symptoms to 'fitten up' with you.

Start with walking, which is a safe, enjoyable and easy way to achieve *basic* fitness. It's cheap, interesting (looking at your surroundings), needs no special clothes except for a comfortable pair of walking shoes, and a big advantage is being able to nose-breathe while doing it.

If you have an aversion to outdoor exercise, hiring or buying an exercycle is a good alternative. Increase cycling times as you would with walking.

Set yourself a time, not distance, to walk (or exercycle). Decide for yourself, based on your symptoms, and err on the light side at first. (Some start as low as three minutes — one and a half minutes out, one and a half back — if walking.)

If you start with walking or cycling times of less than 10 minutes, do two sessions — one in the morning and one in the afternoon — until you can do 10 minutes easily at each session.

At first, limit yourself to walking on the flat. Include hills as you start to feel fitter and more confident. Take smaller strides and *slow down on steep slopes*.

Check that your shoulders and arms are relaxed and loose. Use a good arm swing and walk at a brisk pace.

If you start to feel breathless or experience chest symptoms, 'stop, drop, flop' immediately and take up a rest position — sit on a fence or wall, or stand with your arms on a car roof, partner's shoulders or a fence, and low, slow nose-breathe your way back to normal. Use the Lung Ho salute to check breathing pattern and rate.

Undoubtedly, some days will be harder than others and you must be prepared for ups and downs. Gradually your tolerance to exercise and your ability to control breathing will improve.

When you reach a level where you can walk briskly for 20 minutes every day with slight or no breathless problems, you will have reached a basic level of fitness.

If you are quite happy to keep on with brisk walking, three or four 30-40 minute walks a week are enough to *maintain* basic fitness.

The joys of walking include:

* Aerobic benefits (heart/lung efficiency) are achieved after only 15 minutes of brisk walking.
* Digestion and bowel function are toned up.
* Sleeping patterns improve.
* It is very relaxing.

For variety, include other ways of keeping fit:

* Use the stairs at work. At first, walk up one or down two flights before getting the lift. Increase by one flight a week (to a maximum five up, 10 down).
* Try a rebounder, bouncing to your favourite music.
* Yoga and t'ai chi classes are especially recommended, combining breathing, exercise (especially flexibility) and relaxation.
* Whacking games — tennis, badminton and squash — are good for people who need to release anger or resentments.

• Swimming — you may need extra help with breathing.

Eating and exercise

If you are overweight, regular exercise helps weight loss. Many people mistakenly think that exercise makes you eat more. In fact, you feel less like eating directly after exercise, so if you are trying to lose weight, exercising shortly before meals helps tone down the appetite.

If you are very underweight, take care to avoid heavy-endurance types of exercise, and concentrate on flexibility and low-resistance activities well before meals.

Good nutrition is an important part of fitness. Many authorities cite poor nutrition as a major source of stress. If you have been feeling depressed, not eating properly or getting enough exercise, physical neglect feeds your depression. This drastically increases the potential for sickness and misery.

Skipping meals and relying on 'comfort' foods (chocolate bars) to boost flagging energy levels will only add to an already overburdened nervous system. Hyperventilators tend to interpret their fatigue symptoms as being due to low blood sugar (hypo-glycaemia). But sugar is not, and never has been, an essential part of our diet. The sugar 'high' after eating sweets is short-lived. The body's production of the hormone insulin soon clears the high blood-sugar level and works to restore a normal balance, resulting in a further slump in energy. Reaching for more sugar only repeats the cycle. Choose protein snacks instead — nuts or cheese, for instance — as these keep blood sugar levels steadier longer. For this reason, a high protein diet is recommended for chronic hyperventilators, especially those prone to panic attacks. Experiment and see for yourself.

Alcohol, another high sugar source, tends to accelerate your heart-rate, fuelling HVS. While one glass of wine is an excellent relaxant, more may be asking for trouble.

Smoking

Smoking is another habit that complicates a hyper-ventilator's life. It is not hard to imagine the chaos that strong inhalations of smoke wreak upon your already 'hyper' breathing.

Try to give up smoking while you are retraining your breathing patterns. Join a smoke cessation group. See if you can spot fellow hyperventilators.

Nicotine patches or short, decreasing courses of nicotine chewing gum can help control nasty withdrawal symptoms.

It is usually more difficult to give up the *rituals* of smoking, and for hyperventilators that includes that first quick inhalation after lighting up.

Every time you think of the pleasures of smoking, give equal time to acknowledging the harmful effects and what it is doing to your heart and breathing rates.

Consider whether smoking is an excuse to hyperventilate.

Think about what kind of smoker you are:

- If you smoke to relax, try total body relaxation instead.
- If you smoke to give yourself a lift, get out in the fresh air or do some stretches instead.
- If you smoke because of the ritual of handling cigarettes or other smoking paraphernalia, invest in some worry beads to occupy your hands.

Remember: smoking heavily is asking for trouble. Stopping is best. Cutting down helps.

Regular exercise helps release naturally occurring opiopeptides into the bloodstream, and these make you feel good.

Bones are kept strong too, especially important for post-menopausal women, or those on courses of steroids.

Regular enjoyable exercise builds reserves against HVS. Keeping fit helps conquer panicky feelings. Movement and pleasure in physical action is a very basic human need. Enjoyable exercise is very much part of recovery.

Further reading

Body Sense, Vernon Coleman (Thames and Hudson, London, 1984).

'Hyperventilation Syndrome and Muscle Fatigue', H. Folgering and A. Snik, *Journal of Psychosomatic Research*, vol. 32, no. 2, 1988.

'The Natural Exercise Prescription', Z. Altug and M. Miller, *Clinical Management*, vol. 9, no. 3.

Ten

Rest and sleep

Adequate rest and sleep are vital to good health. One of the most common HVS symptoms people complain of is erratic sleep and vivid or bad dreams. Sound sleep provides a total release from the pressures of daily life. Being deprived of satisfying sleep causes a great deal of distress and anxiety to an already 'stretched' nervous system.

Very few people get through life without experiencing muddled sleep patterns, either from extremes of happiness or despair. Someone newly in love hardly seems to need any sleep at all, and feels no worse for it. But during periods of stress or sickness the body demands more sleep. Anxiety and fear about the symptoms of HVS may be one reason for sleeplessness. But the vivid dreams and nightmares, where the hyperventilator wakes with a pounding heart and a sense of panic, may make sleep itself fearful.

Normal sleep

Sleep is controlled from a regulating centre deep in the brain stem. It processes messages from all over the body — joints, muscles, organs — as well as

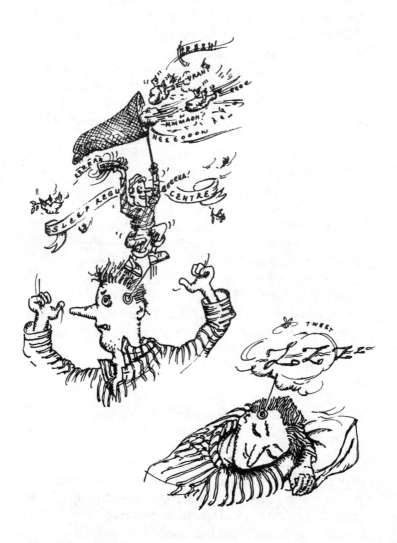

from the higher thought centres in the brain — to either induce sleep (low levels of stimulation to the sleep regulating centre) or wakefulness (high levels of stimulation). So a calm mind as well as a relaxed body is needed for satisfying sleep.

Sleep goes through cycles of quiet sleep, which is true rest with a *quiet* brain. This cycle lasts about an hour. This is followed by rapid eye movement (REM) sleep, a shorter cycle of about 20 to 30 minutes where the brain is very *active*. This is dream-time.

During quiet sleep, the body's metabolic rate, blood pressure and heart rate lower slightly, and the breathing rate is deep and regular. In REM sleep, the heart beats up to 5 per cent faster, there is a slight increase in blood pressure and metabolic rate, the eyes dart about under closed lids, and breathing becomes irregular. The average sleep needed for an adult is seven and a half hours — five complete quiet plus REM sleep cycles. Individual patterns vary widely of course according to age, health and personality.

Why do people with HVS have sleep problems?

For people with HVS, who are sensitive to very small fluctuations in carbon dioxide levels in their blood, the irregular breathing during REM sleep acts on the unconscious mind, producing vivid or nightmarish dreams and lack of satisfying sleep. Another factor is the respiration centre in the brain, which has become accustomed to lower carbon dioxide levels during waking hours. It sends distress signals to the habitual hyperventilator who may be relaxing and breathing 'low and slow' during sleep. Rather like the 'air hunger' sensations felt when starting breathing retraining, the sleeper wakes gasping for air. Stress levels, high enough during waking hours, are added to by disturbed rest and anxiety over poor sleep. But once natural breathing patterns are restored by day natural sleep patterns return at night. For some, this happens quickly. But for others, the downward spiral started by wakefulness, worry, nightmares and sleeplessness often takes time, and a great deal of patience and understanding, to spiral up and away from.

If you are dependent on sleeping pills, the following will be of little use. While sleeping pills are often a blessing for short stressful times, if used continuously for more than two weeks they cease to work effectively. They are addictive. Withdrawal from them must be gradual and undertaken with skilled help. Only use the Good Sleep Plan once you have decided to make a success of getting off the 'little blue pills'.

The Good Sleep Plan

Try these simple strategies, and give yourself time to re-establish a good sleep routine. Let your family and friends know your plans. If you share your bed, your partner will definitely need to know!

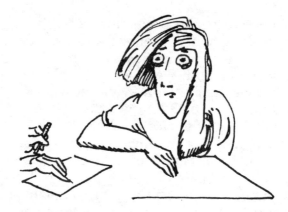

- Make your bedroom a stress-free zone. No television, telephone or noisy clocks.
- Small changes, such as new bed linen or moving the bed, can help start a new routine and break old associations.
- Soft low lighting helps create a restful atmosphere.
- Use the bed for sleeping only.
- No reading, eating, sewing, writing letters, talking on the phone.
- Making love is an exception. Satisfying sex is a powerful prelude to relaxed sleep. Unfortunately, deep post-orgasmic relaxation lasts only four or five minutes, so if you haven't fallen asleep by then it is of no added benefit. Seek expert help if anxiety about sex is a problem.
- Avoid rich, heavy or late-night dinners, or Chinese food (high in monosodium glutamate) at the end of the day.
- Cut out coffee and strong tea for a month. Try decaffeinated. Reintroduce it gradually after a month, and even then, try and avoid it after 4 p.m. If you are a heavy

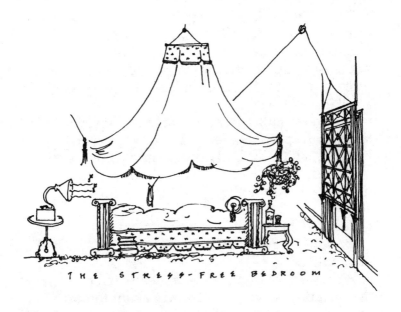

THE STRESS-FREE BEDROOM

coffee drinker, be prepared for withdrawal
symptoms such as irritability and shakiness. Drink
plenty of water.
• Avoid television news and talkback radio for a
month. Watch only light or funny programmes or
videos. Reduce extremes of negative and positive
stimulation three or four hours before sleep.
• Exercise. As noted in Chapter 9, exercise helps
induce sleep — if possible within four or five hours
of bed-time.
• Have a warm bath or shower before going to bed.

Oil of lavender is an age-old remedy for calming and relaxing mind and body. Add drops to the bathwater. For those without a bath, try a few drops on the corner of your pillow.

• Fix a regular time to go to bed and get up in the morning. *Never go to bed earlier or get up later than those appointed times.*

• Cut out day sleeps. Daytime 'tiredness' is more often caused by boredom or lack of activity. Go for a stroll instead of snoozing.

• Try warm milk as a night-cap. Milk has high levels of tryptophanase[*] — a naturally occurring enzyme which the body digests and converts into serotonin. This 'sleep nectar' has a powerful influence in promoting good moods and sound sleep.

• Sedative herb teas such as pasaflora or chamomile are safe alternatives for those who don't like milk.

• Write a list of things to be remembered or done the next day, so you don't worry about tomorrow, today. Constant projecting into the future (or past) is a sure-fire sleep-killer.

• Try to avoid going to bed on an unresolved fight or argument.

---

[*] Tryptophanase has been available in tablet form, and has been used for over 25 years in New Zealand as a non-addictive 'natural' alternative to sleeping pills. Recent research in the US and Europe has shown that high dosages may be linked to a sometimes fatal blood disorder; contaminated stocks are thought to be a possible cause of the problem. While there is doubt, rely on dietary intake of tryptophanase. (Protein foods such as milk, poultry, meat, fish and cheese are rich sources.)

Getting off to sleep

Based on the sleep-retraining method devised by Dr Richard Bootzin of the US, the following regime has proved extremely successful. People who have tried this scheme and stuck to it find it takes between two and six weeks to start working, and feel it is well worth the effort in restoring refreshing drug-free sleep.

- Once prepared and in bed, practise low, slow diaphragmatic breathing (in and out through the nose) and relaxation techniques. Check for tension areas and let them go.
- In a comfortable sleeping position (usually side lying), glance at the time and if after 15 minutes you are still awake, get out of bed. Go into another room and do something else. (Read, watch a funny video, play Patience, listen to soothing music.) When you feel ready to sleep, go back to bed, and if again you are not asleep within 15 minutes, repeat the sequence until you do. Try this approach to early morning waking as well. *Learn to associate bed with sleep — if you're not sleeping, don't stay in bed.*

If your appointed waking time happens to come in the middle of a deep, quiet sleep cycle, you may find it hard to wake up. Don't interpret this as 'waking up tired'.(Many people admit they let this feeling colour their whole day.) It just means you have woken from the Deep Sleep cycle.

If, however, your appointed waking time comes towards the end of REM sleep cycle, you will wake up

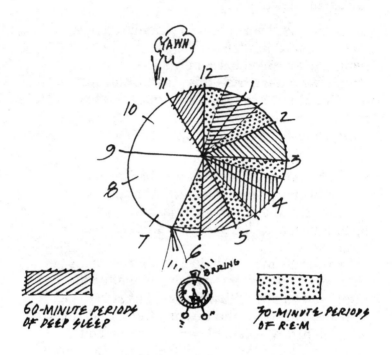

60-MINUTE PERIODS OF DEEP SLEEP

30-MINUTE PERIODS OF R.E.M

more alert and with fleeting memories of dreams. But if nightmares wake you with hyperventilation symptoms, get up and recover in the sitting rest position (see page 55), concentrating totally on relaxing your neck and shoulders, and nose-breathing low and slow. Soothing music helps too. When your breathing is under control and your heart rate has slowed, try going back to sleep, knowing hyperventilation is the problem and you have techniques to combat it.

A large part of success in restoring good sleep patterns is change of attitude. People who go to bed expecting *not* to sleep, are usually proved right.

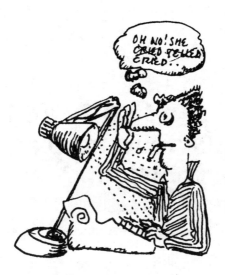

Breathing control and relaxation will remove hyperventilation-induced symptoms.

Your poor sleep pattern can be challenged, and a new refreshing one restored.

A few people never manage to establish 'normal' sleep patterns. If you are a life-long night-owl, at least make it anxiety-free time and use the extra hours of wakefulness creatively and with acceptance.

Further reading

Getting to Sleep, Ellen Mohr Catalauo (New Harbinger Publications, Oakland, 1990).

A Good Night's Sleep, J. S. Maxem (W. W. Norton, New York and London, 1981).

Natural Sleep (How to Get Your Share), P. Goldberg and D. Kaufman (Rodale Press, Emmaus, Pennsylvania, 1978).

Eleven

What can family and friends do to help a hyperventilator?

Learn to be a very good listener.

Always use positive language — 'Let your shoulders go' rather than 'Don't tense your shoulders', or 'Breathe low and slow' instead of 'Don't breathe so fast'. If you meet irritation at your observations, apologise and back off.

Discuss 'flash points' at home or work where tensions are highest, and see if they can be avoided, confronted, or shared.

Use touch instead of words where possible. A gentle massage to tense shoulders may be far better than words. Scalp massages sooth tension headaches and tight scalp muscles. Hand and foot massages are also intensely soothing.

Try not to be over-protective. This can be very difficult, especially with children and teenagers. If

someone close to you is having a bad spell,
remember it's their choice whether to use their new
coping strategies, not yours.

Encourage rest/relaxation times. Hyperventilators
often feel guilty about needing time to relax. Help
them recognise that not only are they helping
themselves, but their family/partner/friends as well.
Join them if you're feeling under strain yourself.

If you live with someone whose self-esteem is
very low and they have become socially isolated, a
gradual re-entry into the outside world is best
initiated by the hyperventilator themselves, as they
start to feel more in control. Realise it may take a
long time. Don't push or nag.

Try to keep stimulation levels down at stressful
times. Be thoughtful about noise and social
pressures. Avoid stressful topics at meal-times.

Above all, be relaxed.

Ideal gifts for a chronic hyperventilator
A sheepskin underlay for the bed.
Worry beads.
Walking shoes.
A funny video.
Oil of lavender.
A course of massages.
A recording of Roger Eno's *Voices.*

Twelve

Last words

A final and encouraging story, from M, a 39-year-old woman with HVS:

Even though on the outside I always looked a fairly laid-back sort of person, I've absorbed an awful lot of stress in my time. About eight or nine years ago I started to be not so . . . resilient.

On the surface I had it all: good marriage, husband a success object, two great kids and an interesting part-time job. Total fulfilment, you'd think. But after a slight accident, when I fell down some steps and had a period of back pain and sleeping badly, I started getting uptight and panicky about minor things. The kids were little then, and I found that pretty stressful. Besides feeling vaguely unwell, I was aware of my breathing — feeling that all the air was pushing up in my chest, trying to stop me breathing. I talked about these symptoms to my doctor. He didn't say much, but when he was out of the room I peeped at his notes and saw that he'd written 'Anxiety attacks' to describe my symptoms. I felt terrible — it reinforced my lack of self-confidence, which was already at an all-time low.

The crunch came a few months later when one day at home, out of the blue, I felt hot and clammy, heart racing and breathless, for no reason. I crawled to bed but felt I couldn't get flat enough; I wanted to press myself on the floor. I managed to telephone my husband and whisper, 'I'm dying' — I really thought I was. The feelings of flying apart, absolute terror, falling down through the world, spinning through the universe . . . was the worst thing I'd ever experienced.

My GP gave me a course of sleeping pills and Oxazepam tranquillisers to take if I had any more 'attacks'. Even though the Oxazepam took 20 minutes to work, I relaxed within two minutes of taking them.

For the last four years I haven't been able to go out without a bottle of Oxazepam in my bag. Over the last year, since starting treatment, I've hardly had to use them. And last week I achieved a major breakthrough: I felt confident enough in my ability to control my breathing to leave the pills at home.

After years of clinging on, being 'clenched' all the time, when you do let go a lot of things happen. After the initial glow of having HVS diagnosed — that there is something wrong and it *can* be fixed — I had a time of feeling worse. I found it really hard learning to relax, to take time for myself and make it a priority. The whole family has had to adapt to these changes.

It's taken about eight months for me to feel that I've recovered. I sleep pretty well now, and I don't panic if I have a bad night. I use visualisations a lot. Before going to sleep I relax by imagining a big soda bottle in my chest, and I slowly unscrew the top, letting out the built-up pressure little by little until it's all gone. By then my breathing is low and slow and I feel good. When I relax lying on my stomach I visualise a nasty little goblin squeezing my upper-back muscles with knobbly hands. I concentrate on those hands and watch them loosen their grip, let go, stop controlling me and disappear. Imagining slowly unravelling a tightly knotted rope is useful when I'm out and about.

I feel really glad not to be dependent on pills any more. I feel better being fitter and having physical reserves again.

Whenever the going gets tough I just think about . . . my next breath!

Conclusion

Hyperventilation Syndrome is alive and thriving in the 1990s. Diagnosis and definition have been contentious issues in recent years and remain the subject of lively debate world-wide, amongst health professionals. However, enough 'sufferers' have responded to physiotherapy treatments involving breathing retraining, relaxation and exercise, and have enjoyed the far-reaching benefits of balanced blood gases and pH levels to make following the BETTER breathing plan a positive option. Fifty per cent of the cure is knowing about and understanding the nature of HVS. The rest is a commitment to restore natural breathing patterns. Remember, it will take time.

To start, work on breathing — pattern first then rate — and relaxation. Tune into your breathing *regularly*, concentrating on 'Lips together, jaw relaxed, breathing low and slow'.

If relaxation seems pointless at first, keep practising. You will soon appreciate the importance of an effective relaxation response.

Organise family and friends so that you can start the sleep regime as soon as possible.

Start exercising only when your breathing is consistently low and slow, and once you have developed a good relaxation response.

Don't make the mistake of trying to achieve fitness too quickly, even if you have been super-fit in the past. The aim of movement and activity is *enjoyment*. Watch out for those aggressive and competitive instincts. Put them 'on hold' for a while.

Restoring normal diaphragmatic breathing may take a long time. Don't be too hard on yourself if you do go off the rails and lapse into disordered 'over-breathing'. Take a break. Use a rest position.

Focus all your attention on breathing, relaxing and reducing lung volumes.

Index